Have You Herb

Stephanie Ham

REJOICE
Essential Publishing

Stephanie Ham/Rejoice Essential Publishing

PO BOX 512

Effingham, SC 29541

www.republishing.org

Unless otherwise indicated, scripture is taken from the King James Version.'

Have You Herb/Stephanie Ham

ISBN-13: 978-1-956775-39-6

Scripture taken from the New King James Version®. Copyright © 1982 by Thomas Nelson. Used by permission. All rights reserved.

Scripture quotations marked (NIV) are taken from the Holy Bible, New International Version®, NIV®. Copyright © 1973, 1978, 1984, 2011 by Biblica, Inc.™ Used by permission of Zondervan. All rights reserved worldwide. www.zondervan.com

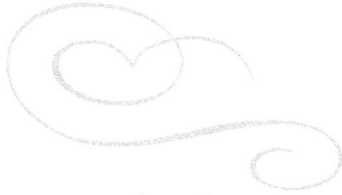

Acknowledgements

IN WRITING THIS BOOK, I have so many people to be thankful for along my journey. God is so phenomenal. He has a way that is mighty sweet. God places you around people that do not mind pushing you into your destiny. For instance, all thanks goes out to my late Apostle Ervin Dease who went on to be with the Lord and his wife, First Lady Mary Dease who is still among the living. They are my spiritual parents from Bennettsville, South Carolina.

I thank my best friend forever (BFF), First Lady Caroline Fletcher-Jackson, and her husband, Lafayette Jackson. They are pastors of Latter Reign Church.

I appreciate Mother Cora Jackson and Elder Nancy Edwards. I am thankful for the whole Dease' family: Junior, Brain and Dee-Dee, Pastor Derrick and Yolanda Dease.

I honor Robin & Mary Fletcher and mother Fletcher, who has gone home to be with the Lord. I want to give a special shout out to Prophetess Teresa Townsend Allen, Minister Janice Morrison, Prophetess Tasha Moses, and Prophet Tron Moses, Shareika Purcell Townsend, Tabitha Quick and a host of spiritual siblings from Solid Rock Holiness Church.

To my mentor team, Kimberly & Tron Moses, God has used you all to push me into my destiny.

To my beautiful family with whom God has blessed me, I am sometimes misunderstood but I love you dearly.

To my husband Leo A. Ham, you stick by my side no matter what we go through.

A special thanks to my four handsome sons: Kayshawn Whack, Obadiah Whack, Yahdiah Ham and stepson Jaleel Scott, and a host of grandbabies Kelsey, Jarineeks, O'So, Tsediah, and a grandbaby I grow to love as my own, Innocence Pratt.

Thanks to my nephews Young Mr. Richards aka Malek Hawkins, King and Baby Jamaica, Lance Ham, Spencer Ham, Chance Ham.

To my beautiful nieces Morgan Harrison, Choice, Brittney, and Ham, thank you.

Also, my sisters-in-law, Suzette Ham, Dentata Ham, Lura Ham, thank you.

Last but not least, my beautiful mom, Deloris Whack-Richards aka Momma-Dee, and my mother-in-law, Mrs. Dorothy Ham, are my ride or die queens and you guys have always kept me uplifted.

CONTENTS

INTRODUCTION..1

CHAPTER 1:   My Testimony.................8

CHAPTER 2:   Sensational Scent Of
Lavandula......................17

CHAPTER 3:   Ingredients....................23

CHAPTER 4:   Let's Take It Back To
Eden Herbalist Style.....28

CHAPTER 5:   Let's Talk About
Hyssop...........................41

CHAPTER 6:   Dandelion......................48

CHAPTER 7:   Red Clover.....................51

CHAPTER 8:   Hyssop...........................53

CHAPTER 9:   Tsediah Essential Oil....55

CHAPTER 10:   Colunga Oil....................57

CHAPTER 11:   Plantain.........................59

CHAPTER 12:   St. John's Wort.............60

CONCLUSION...62

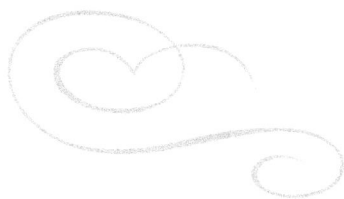

Introduction

Have you herb? One day my husband and I were talking and he came up with the title of this book. I thought it was so cute and it made me chuckle. He knows that I am into herbology and supports my business, "Misfits Forgotten," where I make oils, body products, and smoothies with various herbs. Years ago, I met a herbalist and he taught me the benefits of herbs. I was very sick in my body but followed the regimen he put me on and miraculously was healed. I will share more about this experience later in this book. The topics of herbs may turn off some Christians, but they need to understand that God created herbs. Some medicine that we buy today has extracts from plants, flowers, herbs, etc. If people truly understand that God created herbs for our benefit, there would be less sick-

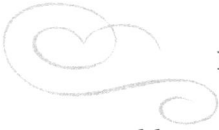

ness and less money spent on drugs. Herbology isn't really taught much in the Christian community and some may call it demonic due to a lack of understanding. When some people don't understand something, especially supernatural things, they call it a demon.

God can heal in every aspect. Ezekiel 47 talks about this. Ezekiel 47:12 (NKJV) says, *"Along the bank of the river, on this side and that, will grow all kinds of trees used for food; their leaves will not wither, and their fruit will not fail. They will bear fruit every month, because their water flows from the sanctuary. Their fruit will be for food, and their leaves for medicine."* As you read this verse, you can see God's plan to use leaves (herbs) for medicine.

In the beginning, God created the heavens and the earth. He also created the plants and flowers we see today. After God created everything, He examined His creation and saw that it was good (Genesis 1). Herbs are God's creation. Also, God told Adam and Eve the things they could and could not eat in the garden of Eden (Genesis 2:16). He knew what was healthy and beneficial for us. Our God is so phenomenal. He had a great purpose when He created man and woman. What if Adam and Eve never sinned? Could you imagine living a long life like Abraham and Sarah? Sin equals death (Romans 6:23) and it shortens our lives.

In the Biblical days, there was no butcher to take meat through the curing process. The people ate bitter herbs that were acidic to purify their bodies. For instance on Passover, they ate lamb with bitter herbs and never got sick. They were healthy. They weren't sick with all the diseases that we have today. However, some people were sick due to disobedience. Some of these diseases did exist in the Biblical days. King David was known to have an STD because he sinned against God. Depending on the translation, Psalm 38:5-7 mentions how his loins were filled with a loathsome disease.

Psalm 38:5-7 (NIV)

⁵ *My wounds fester and are loathsome*
   because of my sinful folly.
⁶ *I am bowed down and brought very low;*
   all day long I go about mourning.

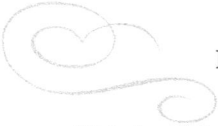

7 My back is filled with searing pain;
   there is no health in my body.
8 I am feeble and utterly crushed;
   I groan in anguish of heart.

Certain diseases can take a toll on your body. You may read about the scabs and scars but might not know what condition they had. However, if you pay attention to the symptoms they mentioned, you will know what disease they were afflicted with due to your medical training or experiences. When you become knowledgeable of certain terms, you are very aware of the people's afflictions in the Bible. Yet, God had herbs available for healing.

However, the enemy comes in and perverts the truth. In other words, the devil twists what God said that was good. Agents of Satan will use herbs for a demonic agenda. However, some believers in Jesus won't use natural remedies for health benefits. This book's objective is to glorify God for His creation and to redeem herbology. I am snatching back this revelation from the enemy and imparting it to you. The enemy is a counterfeit. He takes things and tries to put fear in people so they can be ignorant while never coming into the knowledge of the truth.

God is adamant that we will be in good health, prosper as our soul prospers (3 John 2). One way to be in good health is diet. There is a strong correlation between the foods that we eat and diseases. For instance, if you eat a bunch of fatty foods, you will be at a higher risk of developing diabetes, heart disease, or strokes. God created herbs to be natural remedies for humanity. The western culture depends heavily on the pharmaceutical industry, but in other nations, they have to use what God has given them, which are plants, trees, or herbs.

God works supernaturally. I believe in God's healing power. However, God gives us wisdom and we must be a good steward over our bodies. We only have one body in our earthly lives. When we go to heaven, we will have new glorified bodies (1 Corinthians 15:35-58). So we must take care of our bodies while we are earthen vessels. One way we can do this is to take natural supplements. For instance, during the COVID-19 pandemic, the Lord opened up

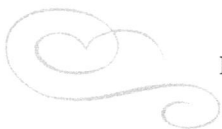

most of the churches' eyes to the importance of herbs. Most discovered that some herbs such as elderberry could build up their immune system, and they began taking a daily supplement.

The pharmacy industry also fights people from trying natural remedies because they will lose money. It's an oxymoron to discover that the same industry trying to fight the average person from using herbs is using it themselves. Some medication may have extracts of different plants inside of it. The pharmaceutical industry always takes credit. Tabitha Brown promotes Goli, a company that makes gummies. These gummies are nothing but herbs. Most people aren't aware of this fact.

We are God's children and He wants the best for us. When God created the earth, He gave us everything that we needed to survive. It's up to us to use these tools. God does heal through herbs. Why are people okay with God healing people through surgery but not herbs? We must renew our minds and stop putting God in a box.

We might be saved, but we need to have a deeper connection with God. Our connection goes beyond our salvation, but we must trust God and believe that He is a healer. Again, God can heal through herbs. In this book, I'll show you how God heals through herbs and the benefit of herbs. Also, I will share my testimony so you can witness God's miraculous healing power through herbs. Lastly, a dictionary will be provided so you can become knowledgeable of the various uses of different herbs. Have you herb?

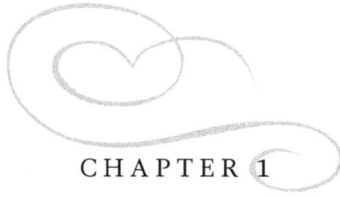

CHAPTER 1

My Testimony

GOD IS A HEALER. I discovered this many years ago when I was a Black Jew. I didn't know that I was deceived and in error. I was sleeping around and became infected with STDs. I didn't know that I was violating my body. Our bodies are the temple of the Holy Spirit (1 Corinthians 6:19). I was going to clubs and sleeping with men because my friends were doing it. I wanted to fit in with the crowd. I was a construction worker and I was dating an older man who was my sugar daddy. He would pay all my bills, so I got to keep my paycheck. He infected me with Syphilis. I had just ended my relationship with Dingo, the stripper. Even though I didn't have a relationship with God during this time, He still extended His beatitude. He still gave me His mercy and grace. God healed my body even when I had done all these horrible things. I was introduced to a herbalist, Atara, who taught me about hyssop, red clover, dandelion, and other herbs.

God's healing virtue can flow through herbs, especially if you take the proper ones for your situation. I am a living witness to how God uses these herbs to take away the sickness and disease that may be plaguing your body. We must eat healthy. The herbalist had me eat a certain way while I took the herbs. It was a routine while I was going through the process. When I woke up in the morning, I would brush my teeth with dandelion because it is a blood purifier, but it also takes away gingivitis or other dental problems. I got the dandelion in the herbal store. You can get it from Amazon as well, and it comes in various forms, such as powder or capsules.

Next, the herbalist had me drink red clover tea two or three times a day. I would eat small portions every two to three hours. In North America, most of us eat big size portions for breakfast, lunch, or dinner. However, I was on a strict regimen. For instance, one portion or meal

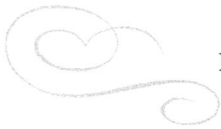

was rolled oats or oatmeal. I would add soymilk, raisins, almonds sometimes. Throughout the day, I would eat dry fruits such as raisins or walnuts. I had to cut out red meats, but I would have lamb. I also would eat turkey and fish. Sometimes, I would have sweet potatoes, salads, and broccoli. I made this a lifestyle and it kept me healthy. It cut down on obesity.

Atara also formulated a tonic, a special drink where he mixed different herbs that I had to drink to purify my blood. These herbs dealt with antiviral infections that cleansed the body from sexual diseases. Atara also showed me which herbs were specialized to heal specific parts of the body. After God healed my body from Syphilis, I had to go through another healing process. It was difficult to conceive a child due to the damage that Syphilis caused to my reproductive organs. Atara taught other women and me to douche with certain herbs. For instance, on Mondays and Tuesdays, we had to douche with one set of herbs. Then on other days, we had to rotate using another herb. This regimen cleaned out my female organs and allowed me to conceive a child. I will develop this regimen to sell in my business, "Misfits Forgottens." Afterward, I started to have many children after months of not being able to conceive. I had multiple miscarriages and couldn't make it to full term. Miraculously, I wasn't on this regimen long. No more than three to six months later, I went to St. Mary's hospital and found out that I was pregnant. Another thing about this regimen is that it increased my libido or sex drive. My second son Obadiah was conceived during this time. Once God had healed me, I never had any more STDs. God kept me all these years.

For seven days at 7 pm, I went through the process of taking bitter herbs mixed with oil. I could not skip a day or I would have to start all over again. I couldn't add anything sweet like honey to ensure my organs were purified. I could not wait for the seventh day to be done with the regimen.

I cannot remember which was worse, the shots or the herbs but following the instructions was important. I recall Atara saying the western belief concerning herbs is to think they do not work, but in all reality, it does. Herbs are used a

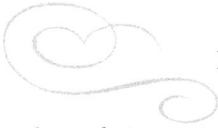

lot of times in the medicine we use. We aren't aware of the name, especially if you're not in the nursing field. For example, research has shown that the mold that produces penicillin can grow on the leaf of Hyssop.[1]

My next step was to continue to eat healthily so my blood won't be contaminated. I could not eat red meat such as beef or pork. Only on Passover I could eat lamb and bitter herbs. I scheduled a doctor's appointment within three to six months to do a new blood test. When the results came back, the doctor was shocked because most people couldn't get rid of the type of STD I had contracted. When the results came back, he ordered another set to ensure there was no mistake. The doctor examined me and took cultures to see any signs of sores, chancre, or palmar lesion on my tongue, hands, feet, and vaginal opening. All cultures came back NEGATIVE. My doctor was so amazed that he had other doctors examine me and when they checked, they shook their heads, saying, "We can't find anything."

---

1. "Hyssop." Herbal Encyclopedia, December 24, 2010. https://www.cloverleaffarmherbs.com/hyssop/.

God can do exceedingly abundantly above all we can ask or think (Ephesians 3:20). To God be all the Glory! HALLELUJAH, THANK YOU, JESUS. MY LORD, WON'T HE DO IT! God made a believer out of me. I have seen with my eyes what the Power of God can do. I am so overwhelmed with His Love And the Power of the Holy Spirit.

God cleaned me up and I have been made whole ever since. I have seen the hands of God moving in the healing business. God has used the Herbalist Atrata mighty with movie stars. May God bless his legacy. God has used Dr. Sebi to heal millions of people across the world. Dr. Sebi was asked to prove all the people he had healed from Aids. There were so many who showed up in the courtroom that they threw the case out because he had proven it to be true.

If the pharmaceutical companies have not discovered, developed medications, then they believe that the symptoms are not curable.

God has a way that is mighty sweet. Since Co-vid-19, several doctors have spoken out about

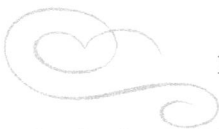

herbs beneficial to the body's healing. For instance, one of my doctors, doctor Charles works as a Chiropractor and Nerve Neuropathy. He uses holistic herbs to reverse nerve damage and believes it can be changed through the proper diet. Dr. Charles also wrote a book about it. When stepping out in using herbal products, the only thing is that most insurance does not cover the cost and can sometimes be very expensive. Nevertheless, some doctors do offer a payment plan.

Dr. Pepe Ramnath is an international doctor who speaks on how we need to take care of our bodies by building our immune systems with herbs. He is a spiritual son of Dr. Myles Munroe. I came across an interesting video on Facebook with Dr. Pepe Ramnath and Dr. Rossi Ishmael Khan. This interview discussed what happens when a virus gets in the blood and releases toxins. Derek Oldenkamp, a Doctor of Chiropractic, Doctor Oz, and Doctor Josh Axe are speaking on herbs.

Another powerful healing testimony is of the Gospel singer, Dewayne Woods. He was raised as a Christian but backslid. He started dating a girl and having unprotected sex. He started to get sick and then passed out. One day in 1992, he went to the doctor for a physical and when he went back the next week, they told him that he had HIV. He went to a herbalist and took the prescribed regimen while taking the standard treatment for HIV through the pharmaceutical industry. The power of God flowed through him through the herbs. Years after taking various treatments and seeking God, he was healed. They took him before a national board and did a series of tests and they couldn't find any traces of HIV. He had to keep going back to the doctor for a whole year to confirm these results. So when people say that he was in remission where the symptoms go dormant for a while, he testifies of God's healing power.

We can trust God for our healing. He was with us before the beginning of time and He will be with us until the end of age. When we came out of our mother's womb, God had angels assigned to protect us. When we became saved and got closer to God, we started to hear His voice and learned how to follow His instruc-

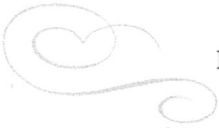

tions. God can still heal you if you have been abused, raped, molested, and gotten a sexual disease. We have to seek God and His wisdom. The medication from the doctors only treated the symptoms while never healing the root of the problem. Only the power of God and His herbs can heal. By Jesus' stripes, we are now healed (Isaiah 53:5).

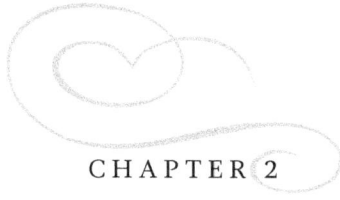

CHAPTER 2

Sensational Scent Of Lavandula

WHAT IS LAVANDULA?

ACCORDING TO ASK A Prepper, it is a sensational scent of lavender that belongs Lamiaceae or mint family. It has many different names, such as garden lavender, true lavender, narrow-leaved lavender, English lavender, and common lavender. This plant has been around for many years and navigated across France, Spain, and the Mediterranean. Most of our lavender plant

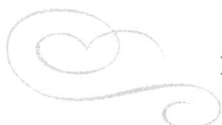

comes from Europe. There are over 40 different colors of purples and a few kinds of Lavandula.[2]

1.   Where does it grow?

Let us start with the Spanish Lavender flower, Lavandula Stoechas, also known as Topped lavender. It grows in late spring and early summer. Its colors are mainly pink to purple. In the photo below, you can see the spikes, which are around 2 cm long. The leafless stems are 10–30 cm (4–12 in) long and open with an upside-down heart with five teeth. This flower appears as a bright velvet purplish color; depending on the climate, it grows to be about 30-100 cm tall.[3]

2.   Where does it grow?

Below is a photo of Lavandula pedunculata, or French Lavender. According to Wikipedia, it can be found in several Mediterranean countries, including France, Spain, Portugal, Italy,

2. Heather. "Ask A Prepper." Ask a Prepper, February 18, 2022. https://www.askaprepper.com/.
3. "Lavandula Stoechas." Wikipedia. Wikimedia Foundation, July 3, 2022. https://en.wikipedia.org/wiki/Lavandula_stoechas#:~:text=Lavandula%20stoechas%2C%20the%20Spanish%20lavender,%2C%20Portugal%2C%20Italy%20and%20Greece.

and Greece.[4] It is known for its butterfly-like, narrow petals that emerge from the top of its narrow stalk. The Aromatic smell is distinctive and leaves you coming back for more. By the way, it loves a hot climate. It stands about 24 in. (60cm). Fall colors are gray-green with a round dark plumpish purple.

3. Where does it grow?

Lavandula lanata, the woolly lavender, is native to southern Spain. According to Wikipedia, it has an evergreen dwarf shrub growing to 1 m (3.3 ft) tall and broad. It is noted for the pronounced silver woolly hairs on its leaves. The deep violet-purple flowers are borne on narrow spikes. The extraordinarily strong fragrance is powerful in attacking and killing fungal disease. This plant grows July- September. Bees, birds, butterflies love it for the many benefits.[5]

---

4. "Lavandula Pedunculata." Wikipedia. Wikimedia Foundation, January 3, 2022. https://en.wikipedia.org/wiki/Lavandula_pedunculata.

5. "Lavandula Lanata." Wikipedia. Wikimedia Foundation, January 3, 2022. https://en.wikipedia.org/wiki/Lavandula_lanata#:~:text=Lavandula%20lanata%2C%20the%20woolly%20lavender,the%20Latin%20specific%20epithet%20lanata.

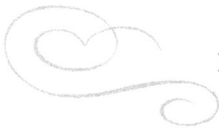

4. Where does it grow?

Lavandula dentata, fringed lavender or French lavender, is native to the Mediterranean, the Atlantic islands and the Arabian Peninsula. According to Wikipedia, it grows to 60 cm (24 in) tall, it has gray-green, linear, or lance-shaped leaves with toothed edges and a lightly woolly texture. The long-lasting, narrow spikes of purple flowers, topped with pale violet bracts, first appear in late spring.[6]

4. And what is it good for?

I use the organic Lavandula Angustifolia because the leaves are entirely very thin and when it is fully grown, it stands about 1to 3' (0.3m to 0.9 meters). And (1 1/2 inches long 3.75 Cm). (Dr. Nicole Aphelian). Popular places where this plant is found are in the Mediterranean or dry summer climate. When you open a bag of lavender, you will be awakened by the Sensational fresh scent. The aroma is why the bees, birds, and butterflies keep coming back for more.

---

6. "Lavandula Dentata." Wikipedia. Wikimedia Foundation, July 3, 2022. https://en.wikipedia.org/wiki/Lavandula_dentata.

There are three beneficial uses of this herb: edible, medical, and aromatherapy. When ingesting lavender, please research which type is good for culinary. The flowers can be added to ice creams, jams, and vinegar as a flavoring for your salad. Drink as a tincture or tea.

The medical use of lavender is anti-anxiety, diuretic, antiseptic, antispasmodic, and bile-producing. It can help relieve some respiratory, and urinary tract infections, lower blood pressure, asthma, and bronchitis.

Lastly, aromatherapy lavender is important for relaxing, smoothing the body, calming from stress, headaches, and pain relief.

Is lavender found in the Bible anywhere? Yes Absolutely! Lavandula or Lavender was known by a different name, such as Spikenard, and Nard. The nard is a perennial herb with strong, pleasantly scented roots. It is native to high altitudes in the Himalayas, and its range extends from there into western Asia. The roots and spike-like wooly young stems are dried before the leaves unfold and are used for making perfume. It is

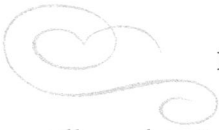

still used in India as a perfume for hair. There is every reason to believe that the spikenard of Scripture (Sg 1:12; 4:13, 14; Mk 14:3; Jn 12:3) came originally from India. Because of the long-distance from which it had to be imported it would be understandably expensive. The best spikenard ointment was commonly imported and sealed in boxes of alabaster, which were stored and opened only on incredibly special occasions.

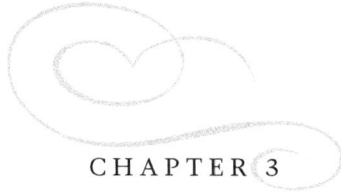

CHAPTER 3

Ingredients

- Various spices were used in the manufacturing of ointments and perfumes:
- aloes (Psalm 45:8; John 19:39);
- balsam (Exodus 30:23; 2 Chronicles 9:1);
- galbanum (Exodus 30:34),
- myrrh, or more literally mastic or ladanum (Genesis 37:25; Genesis 43:11);
- myrrh (Esther 2:12; Matthew 2:11),
- nard (Song of. Sol. Matthew 4:13-14; Mark 14:3; KJV: "spikenard"),
- frankincense (KJV: "incense"; Isaiah 60:6; Matthew 2:11);
- balsam or balm (Genesis 37:25; Jeremiah 8:22);
- cassia (Exodus 30:24; Ezekiel 27:19),
- calamus (Exodus 30:23; Song of Solomon 4:14; NRSV: "aromatic cane"),

- cinnamon (Exodus 30:23; Revelation 18:13),
- stacte (Exodus 30:34),
- onycha (Exodus 30:34).

Onycha is an ingredient derived from mollusks found in the Red Sea, was used in the mixture to be burned on the altar of incense. These spices were used as fragrant incense in worship. They were also mixed with oil to produce the holy anointing oil and to produce cosmetics and medicine.

Apostle Paul may or may not have used Lavandula or " Spikenard Oils" for his handkerchief but he already knew how important it was for the sweet smell of fragrance. He writes about it in 2 Corinthians 2:14–16 (KJV 1900): *14 Now thanks be unto God, which always caused us to triumph in Christ, and makes manifest the savor of his knowledge by us in every place. 15 For we are unto God a sweet savor of Christ, in them that are saved, and in them, that perish: 16 To the one we are the savor of death unto death; and to the other the savor of life unto life. And who is sufficient for these things?*

Apostle Paul would use this pleasant smell of fragrance perfume because they were consecrated for prayer, healing, and worshipping God. All throughout the Bible, some plants were used for prayer, healing, and deliverance. King Solomon, the son of David, wrote a poem about what the sweet-smelling fragrance meant to him.

Mary, are you going to waste oil that you could sell? "I am going to anoint my Master's feet."

MARY OF BETHANY & SPIKENARD OIL: "Lavandula." One of Scripture's most poignant, bittersweet scenes [Mat. 26:6-13; Mark 14:3-9; John 12:3-5] memorializes Mary of Bethany: A woman with an alabaster jar filled with awfully expensive perfume (pure spikenard oil worth an average laborer's annual wage) approaches Yeshua, breaks the jar, and begins pouring the precious oil over His head and feet. As the house fills with the oil's pungent fragrance, the Lord says to those nearby: "She has done a beautiful thing for me. She poured this perfume on me to prepare my body for burial. I tell you that through-

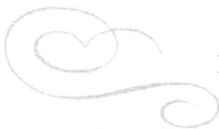

out the whole world, what she has done will be told in her memory." Obviously, our Lord was deeply touched by Mary's unselfish, thoughtful, heartfelt, sacrificial expression of devotion and profound love. Some Bible commentators deem Mary's faithful act as the utmost example of what God desires in believers.[7]

Song of Solomon 4:13-16 says, *"[13] Thy plants are an orchard of pomegranates, with pleasant fruits; camphire, with spikenard,[14] Spikenard and saffron; calamus and cinnamon, with all trees of frankincense; myrrh and aloes, with all the chief spices: [15] A fountain of gardens, a well of living waters, and streams from Lebanon.[16] Awake, O north wind; and come, thou south; blow upon my garden, that the spices thereof may flow out. Let my beloved come into his garden, and eat his pleasant fruits."*

King Solomon recites poetry about the sweet fragrance for the one he loved. The fountain of the garden speaks life and produces fruit which is the Holy Spirit. Jesus Christ's fresh fragrance enters your nostrils.

---

7. "Anointing Oil." Anointing Oil Teaching. Accessed July 31, 2022. https://www.abbaoil.com/t-anointingoilteaching.aspx.

David says, "Taste and see that the Lord is good." Jesus pours His love upon you and purifies you from the inside out.

King Solomon is speaking about the Holy Spirit. When Jesus stepped inside a room, the atmosphere changes. He says his sweet aroma is a fragrance that filled the temple from the North, South, East, and West.

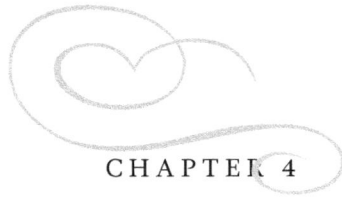

CHAPTER 4

Let's Take It Back To Eden Herbalist Style

HERE IS A LIST OF HERBS!!!

GOD GAVE THESE INSTRUCTIONS to help heal, deliver, and set the children of Israel free from whatever captivity they were facing.

God has given me a passion for herbs and blessed me with my own business, "Misfit Forgottens," to help others build up their inner and outer immunity system.

Elderberry Blast is one of my top-selling products. Elderberry Blast helps treat cold and flu symptoms. It must be kept in the refrigerator but used within six months. This plant contains many antioxidants that give the berries blue or purple colors. Antioxidants help boost the immune system. Additionally, elderberry blast contains anthocyanins that have anti-inflammatory properties, which may aid in the treatment of arthritis and other chronic disorders. Historically, Native Americans used this plant in tea to treat fevers, coughs, and pain.

The herbs that God spoke to me about using to help benefit the body are rose hip, Vitamins C, D, B6, B12, raw honey, cinnamon, ginger, and echinacea. For pregnant women, I will be adding Red Raspberry Mother's Best.

ELDERBERRY

It can be used for medicinal use. The flowers, leaves, and cooked berries are all useful. I use elderberry berry tincture once a day as a preventative during flu season. It strengthens the immune system, especially if you are travel-

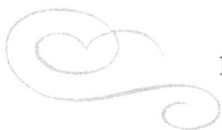

ing. Elderberries have long been recognized as a therapy for a variety of illnesses. You can take it 3x per day if you feel a cold or flu coming. Taking blue elderberry early reduces the chance of catching a cold or the flu. When taken after a flu infection, it reduces the spread of the disease throughout the body and lessens the severity and duration of the virus. Blue elderberry is one of the best anti-viral. There has been much research supporting its effectiveness. It is deemed safe for children. Elderberry is also good for bruised tissue, muscle sprains, and hemorrhoids.

ELDERBERRY FLOWER

This flower helps with eye irritation and conjunctivitis. Elderberry flower tea makes a gentle eyewash and strengthens the immune system. Elderberries have long been recognized as a therapy for a variety of illnesses. It is thought that their beneficial effects are due to their ability to strengthen the immune system[8].

---

8. Apelian, Nicole, and Claude Davis. The Lost Book of Herbal Remedies: The Healing Power of Plant Medicine. United States?: Global Brothers SRL, 2021.

Sea moss/ Bladderwrack: some call it Irish moss. This herb contains 92 of 102 minerals that are in our body. It is a very awesome source to use. It has zinc, calcium, iron, copper, fiber, vitamins, and minerals. Compounding bladderwrack with sea moss builds your metabolism, relieves joint pain and heals the digestive tract.

Sarsaparilla: helps with joint pains, congestive heart failure, high blood pressure, premenstrual syndrome (PMS), nervous system disorders, and urinary problems. It is an Anti-inflammatory and antioxidant.

Soursop: Soursop is beneficial to enhance the skin, nails, and hair. It may help with killing cancer cells and inflammation.

Turmeric: is helpful for a healthy liver. It stimulates natural bowel movements and cleans the gallbladder against stones. It keeps your blood purified.

Yellow dock: It has a good amount of iron to help treat the body from all sexually transmitted diseases and arthritis.

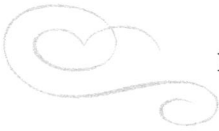

Cannabis: This plant gets such a bad name, but it has a lot of medicinal benefits such as being an anti-inflammatory, relieving chronic pain, helping fight cancer, depression, autism, controlling seizures, ADHD/ADD, and glaucoma. It can slow down Alzheimer's disease.

STAR ANISE

According to Master class, anise has a strong licorice flavor. It is an important commercial fruit worldwide, but mainly in Asia, where most of its market is located. Star Anise has long been used in Asia to help promote good digestion. Its warming flavor and calming influence on digestion make it a wonderful addition to herbal teas targeting digestive wellness as well as respiratory health.[9]

The Autoimmune Protocol states, "Star anise contains anti-inflammatory properties, along with many other therapeutic actions to help promote bodily health. Star anise contains many phytochemicals that act as powerful antioxi-

9. "MasterClass Online Classes." MasterClass. Accessed July 31, 2022. http://www.masterclass.com/.

dants. These phytochemicals are highly inflammatory. In addition to their antioxidant properties, star anise has been a coveted spice for centuries. It has been used for conditions ranging from fighting various cancer, bone health and sleep aid. Star anise, cinnamon, and clove tincture create a powerful immune-strengthening and inflammation-fighting remedy."

Anise

Woe unto you, scribes and Pharisees, hypocrites! for ye pay tithe of mint and anise and cumin, and have omitted the weightier matters of the law, judgment, mercy, and faith: these ought ye to have done, and not to leave the other undone (Matthew 23:23).

Echinacea

This herb modulates the body's natural immune system, encouraging it to operate more efficiently. It raises the body's resistance to bacterial and viral infections by stimulating the immune system.

It also has anti-inflammatory and pain-relieving functions. The anti-microbial and anti-inflammatory effects of echinacea make it an ideal choice for treating urinary tract infections. It is a standard UTI treatment and is often combined with goldenseal root. Echinacea is known to reduce the impact of the common cold and the flu. People who begin taking echinacea extract or tea immediately upon feeling sick heal much more quickly than those who do not. In general, people who take echinacea get well up to four days faster.

Echinacea helps to relieve allergies by stimulating and balancing the immune system. It is especially helpful in relieving asthma attacks. While it does not cure asthma, it reduces the severity of the attack and helps the patient get over attacks. It is also useful for treating bronchitis.

Goldenseal

Goldenseal boosts the effects of many other herbs. Goldenseal reduces irritation and inflammation of the mucous membranes, making it an ideal addition for treating respiratory problems. It is also anti-microbial and anti-viral. Its efficacy is well established for colds, the flu, and other respiratory problems. The anti-microbial properties of goldenseal root are effective against many bacterial infections, including vaginal infections, infectious diarrhea, colds, flu, eye infections, and urinary tract infections.

Cinnamon

According to The Lost Book Of Herbals Remedy, cinnamon can be used for medicinal use and preventative care. The commonly suggested dose for "true cinnamon" (Ceylon) is 1-2 grams with each meal. You can add it to a smoothie or food or use it in tea. Cinnamon improves insulin sensitivity, a key hormone in regulating metabolism and blood sugar. In some metabolic conditions, the body may become insulin resistant. By increasing insulin sensitivity, cinnamon lowers blood sugar levels and helps prevent or treat diabetes. Additionally, cinnamon decreases the amount of glucose that enters your bloodstream after a meal. It slows the breakdown of carbohydrates and prevents blood sugar spikes. Another compound in cinnamon acts like insulin to improve glucose uptake in the cells. Care is needed as cinnamon may cause blood sugar levels to drop too low. 1 to 6 grams of cinnamon lowers triglycerides and "bad" LDL cholesterol.

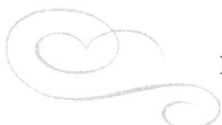

Ceylon Cinnamon works better than Cinnamon sticks because it focuses on correcting diabetes and bad LDL cholesterol.

Cinnamon

Take the following fine spices: 500 shekels of liquid myrrh, half as much of fragrant cinnamon, 250 shekels of fragrant calamus (Exodus 30:23 KJV).

Mullein

According to The Lost Book Of Herbals Remedies, the leaves and flowers of mullein are anti-inflammatory, antiseptic, antispasmodic, astringent, demulcent, diuretic, emollient, expectorant, anodyne (pain-killing), and vulnerary (wound healing). Mullein is a commonly used herbal remedy if you suffer from bronchitis, emphysema, laryngitis, tracheitis, asthma, and tuberculosis. I value it for its efficacy in treating chest complaints such as bronchitis, tuberculosis, and asthma. It reduces oils also. It is an antibacterial that helps prevent infection and speeds healing. Mullein helps to kill the virus to the roots and remove the wart. The juice of the plant can also be used for cramps and muscle spasms.

Raw Honey

Honey contains many medicinal qualities taken from the flower. Once the honey has been cooked or diluted, these properties may no longer exist in beneficial quantities. I prefer to use undiluted raw honey, as it contains pollen and parts of the waxen honeycomb. Honey has a rich medicinal history. It has been used since ancient times to dress wounds and as a cough suppressant.

It can be used for burns and wound healing because of its antibacterial and anti-inflammatory properties. It can be used on diabetic foot ulcers and other skin conditions such as psoriasis and herpes. You can apply it directly to the skin or apply it to the bandage before use. For difficult infections and ulcers, the use of Manuka honey is recommended. Honey lowers blood pressure. When used moderately, in place of sugar, honey may help lower blood pressure. Because of its antioxidant compounds, modest blood pressure reductions can occur when reducing sugar use

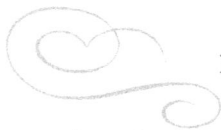

and replacing it with a small amount of honey. Instead of sucrose, honey is made up of glucose and fructose and has a lower glycemic index than sugar. Honey can lower cholesterol and triglycerides. High LDL cholesterol is a strong risk factor for heart disease and plays a major role in atherosclerosis. Honey can improve cholesterol levels.

Never give raw honey to an infant or child under one. Their immature immune systems cannot handle the botulism spores, where older children and adults have a natural immunity (The Lost Book Of Herbals Remedy).

You can take this before or after each meal two to three times a day if your sugar is low. It would be best if you used it in moderation. Always check and monitor while God heals and restores your health.

Cloves

Cloves contain a chemical that protects against age-related cell damage resulting in cancerous changes to your cells. This chemical (eugenol) is also found in basil, cinnamon, and bay leaves (Lost Book Of Disease).

Aloe Vera

Aloe Vera gel is the gelatinous substance inside the leaf. It is used to relieve sunburn, wounds, and other minor skin irritations. It also has internal uses. The gel can be unpleasant and bitter when taken alone. Consuming 1 to 3 ounces (28g to 85g) of aloe vera gel with each meal reduces the severity of acid reflux and the associated heartburn. It also helps the cramping, abdominal pain, flatulence, and bloating. Aloe Vera extract makes a safe and effective mouthwash that reduces swelling, soothes, and provides relief from bleeding or swollen gums. You can rinse with the gel swishing it around, holding it in the mouth for a minute, then spitting it out. If you have type 2 diabetes, you can regulate your blood sugar levels by simply ingesting two tablespoons of Aloe Vera juice or pulp extract daily. I use Aloe Vera inside my smoothie with plenty of fruits and vegetables. I use fresh Aloe Vera or the Aloe Vera Juice with two drops of Elderberry Blast. It does the body wonders.

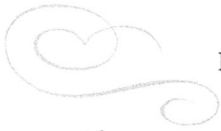

Aloes

He was accompanied by Nicodemus, the man who earlier had visited Jesus at night. Nicodemus brought a mixture of myrrh and aloes, about seventy-five pounds (John 19:39 KJV).

Garlic

Garlic has been used as food and medicine in many cultures for thousands of years, dating back to when the Egyptian pyramids were built.

Garlic today boosts the immune system and helps prevent heart disease. It also helps the effects on hypertension and high cholesterol. Consuming garlic will guard against cancer cell formation in the body. It has a way of reversing numerous diseases.

We remember the free fish we ate in Egypt, along with the cucumbers, melons, leeks, onions, and garlic (Numbers 11:5 KJV).

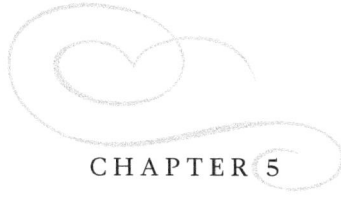

CHAPTER 5

Let's Talk About Hyssop

W**HAT DOES WEBSTER'S DIC-TIONARY** say about hyssop? Is hyssop known by a different name? In Hebrew, hyssop is ezob and in Arabic, zufa. The Greek translation is hyssopos, which refers to a small bush. Hyssop must have been very abundant in Israel as it is mentioned frequently in the Bible (Ex. 12:22; Lv. 14:4, 6, 49, 51; Nm. 19:6; Psalm 51:7; Acts. 9:19; etc.).[10]

What does the Bible say about hyssop?

10. "A Bridge in Europe between Evangelicals and All of Society." Evangelical Focus, August 1, 2022. https://evangelicalfocus.com/.

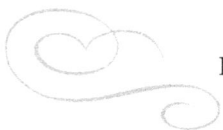

The Bible shows us that hyssop was used for many different beneficial factors, such as medical healing from leprosy, cleansing, purification, and sacrifices.

How many names does hyssop have?

Identification: Anise hyssop grows from 2 to 5 feet (0.6 to 1.5m) tall, with bright green leaves notched at the edge and covered with fine white hairs on the underside. New growth has a purple tint. The plant has an aroma suggestive of mint and anise. The herb is partially woody with branched and usually hairless stems. The fibrous roots are also branching. Clusters of small lilac-blue flowers appear on elongated flower spikes from July through September.

Edible Use: Anise hyssop can be used as a sweetener and to make tea. It can be used as a flavoring or seasoning. The leaves and flowers can be eaten fresh, cooked, or dried.

Medicinal Use: For Heart Health and Angina Pain. An infusion of anise hyssop is a tonic for the heart and a quick remedy for angina pain.

Sores, Wounds, and Burns: For skin infections, wounds, and burned skin, use a poultice of anise hyssop leaves. Soak dried leaves or bruise fresh leaves and flowers and apply them directly to the affected area. Cover with a clean cloth. Anise hyssop leaves have anti-bacterial and antiviral properties.

Facilitates Digestion: Drinking Anise Hyssop Tea with meals eases digestion and prevents excessive gas and bloating.

Diarrhea: Anise hyssop tea helps relieve diarrhea. The tea works best if continued throughout the day, even after the diarrhea has been successfully eliminated. Continuing to sip occasionally prevents the return of diarrhea.

Sore Muscles and Anxiety: Try gathering 3 to 4 tablespoons of anise hyssop leaves in a square of cheesecloth and hang it from the faucet while drawing a bath. The scent released as the water flows calms the spirit. When the bath is ready, drop the herbs into the bathwater and soak your sore muscles in the tub.

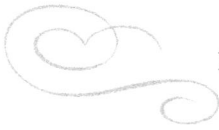

Colds, Flu, Bronchial Congestion: Anise hyssop tea helps expel mucus from the lungs, making it a good choice for treating colds, flu, and congestion.

Herpes: Try Anise Hyssop Essential Oil externally as an antiviral treatment for Herpes Simplex I and II and drink the tea to treat the virus internally.

Poison Ivy: Wash the skin in Anise Hyssop Infusion to help relieve the itchiness of poison ivy.

Athlete's Foot, Fungal Skin Infections, Yeast Overgrowth: Soak the foot or infected area in a bath with a strong infusion of Anise Hyssop. Soak daily until the infection is cured.

Recipes: Anise Hyssop Tea or Infusion. You'll need one cup of boiling water and raw honey to your liking. Add one teaspoon of dried leaves and flowers or one tablespoon of fresh leaves and flowers. Add them to the boiling water and cover tightly. Allow the leaves to steep for 15 minutes.

Where can you find hyssop in the Bible?

Chronic pain: can last for years and range from mild to severe on any given day. It is fairly common, affecting the back, neck, knee, and many other body parts. Hyssop is so magnificent that it cleanses and purifies the body. It helps with gout, joint pain, and poor circulation.

Acute to Chronic: My Tsediah Skincare products are made with Calendula & Lavender and mixed essential oils and can be used all over the body. It is excellent at relieving various external conditions and skin diseases such as eczema and acne. It reduces inflammation, relieves pain, swelling, blemish, scars, diaper rash, skin irritation, anti-fungal, athletic foot, alopecia, and ringworms.

I am so grateful that God Is our Healer from all things:

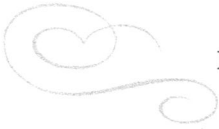

Romans 5:3-5

³ And not only that, but we also glory in tribulations, knowing that tribulation produces perseverance;

⁴ and perseverance, character; and character, hope.

⁵ Now hope does not disappoint, because the love of God has been poured out in our hearts by the Holy Spirit who was given to us.

Ecclesiastes 3:1-4 (NKJV)

¹ To everything there is a season, A time for every purpose under heaven:

² A time to be born, And a time to die; A time to plant, And a time to pluck what is planted;

³ A time to kill, And a time to heal; A time to break down, And a time to build up;

⁴ A time to weep, And a time to laugh; A time to mourn, And a time to dance.

1 Peter 1:6-7 (NKJV)

⁶ In this you greatly rejoice, though now for a little while, if need be, you have been grieved by various trials,

⁷ that the genuineness of your faith, being much more precious than gold that perishes, though it is tested by fire, may be found to praise, honor, and glory at the revelation of Jesus Christ.

Romans 8:28 (NKJV)

And we know that all things work together for good to those who love God, to those who are the called according to His purpose.

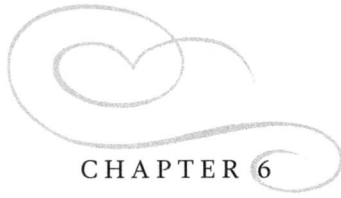

CHAPTER 6

Dandelion

ACCORDING TO THE "LOST Book of Remedies," dandelion is a blood purifier that grows in North America. It extends from detachable plants that reaches deep down into the soil. The plant grows up to a foot and blossoms. The best time to buy the herb is from April to June. This herb has medicinal use such as gastritis, liver problems, skincare, especially warts, treats blood sugar. Dandelion has several beneficial effects on diabetes. Dandelion juice stimulates the production of insulin made in the pancreas, which helps regulate blood sugar levels. It prevents dangerous blood sugar spikes. It helps remove excess sugar from the body. Dandelion also controls lipid levels. Dandelion also prevents and treats certain cancers. Dandelion can be combined with many other herbs, such as burdock root, to fight cancer. Dandelion treats hypertension, boosts your immune system, treats inflammation and arthritis. Dandelion also builds up blood cells.

Dandelion root can be used when dried as a coffee substitute. The root can be cooked and eaten. Even though they are bitter, it tastes similar to turnips. Dandelion flower makes an excellent salad garnish. It can also be battered and fried. Dandelion is bitter when it's in tea form, but you can add some honey to it.

Atari had me brush my teeth with dandelion. It is good to heal gingivitis and bad breath. I felt a difference when I used it. I used to gargle with dandelion and my breath was so fresh. My teeth didn't have any plaque on them. I would use dandelion once a day in the morning. However, it can be used two to three times a day, especially after they eat. I would also use dandelion with other herbs to combat the other bitter-tasting herbs. Some herbs I had to take in their natural form without adding any sugar or honey. You can get dandelions from Amazon or a potential

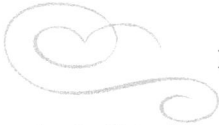

herbalist. You can buy the dandelion in many different forms, such as powder or tea. I used the powder to brush my teeth. You can buy the tea at Walmart or any grocery store. Some forms of dandelion last longer, such as dried, capsules, or teas, compared to the fresh version. I love purchasing herbs from Pacific Botanicals. They are located at 4840 Fish Hatchery Rd, Grants Pass, OR 97527. Their herbs are fresh and well kept. They put invaluable time. You can also order fresh during harvest time. I love to also order from Star West Botanicals.

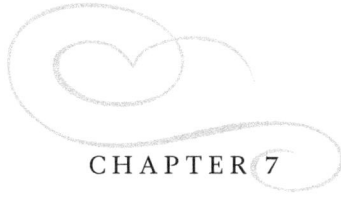

CHAPTER 7

Red Clover

RED CLOVER IS A blood purifier. It relieves symptoms of menopause and is great for cardiovascular health. Red clover increases the HDLs, so it protects against heart disease. Red clover helps with pre and post-menopausal symptoms. It helps regulate your hormones. Red clover is good for skin conditions, including eczema or skin irritation. It is a healing herb, but it heals the inner and outer man. The outer immune system, such as your skin and pores has to be treated as well. The internal immune system includes the blood cells.

Cloves are different from red clover because you bake or cook with it. Cloves are placed inside ham then baked. I also put some in elderberry

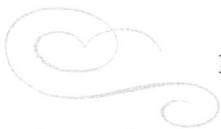

blast when I make it. Cloves aren't bitter, but it has a similar taste to anise or cinnamon. Even though red clover does the same job as dandelion, it's not as bitter. You can cook with red clover and put it in soups and salads. I would drink red clover tea and add some honey to it. Dealing with herbs is a lifestyle. This lifestyle encourages you to eat healthier. When taking herbs, you can't eat two big macs, fries, and a large Dr. Pepper or Sprite. It will defeat the purpose.

I was first introduced to Red Clover in the 90s when Atari showed what it was. I would take red clover in the afternoon or close to going to bed because it relaxes you.

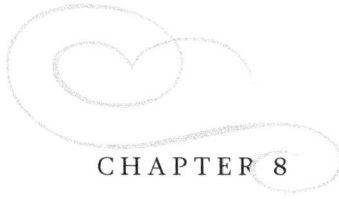

CHAPTER 8

Hyssop

YSSOP IS A BLOOD purifier. It has been around for centuries. It's in the herb family with medicinal factors. The Hebrews used it during ceremonies or sacrificing animals. The Old Testament and Old Testaments used it. Hyssop and vinegar were put on a sponge to give to Jesus. King David speaks about hyssops in Psalms 51. Lord wash me with hyssop and make me white as snow. He prayed these prayers after he committed adultery. David used certain herbs to treat the STD that he had gotten from sexual sin. He repented after suffering and was healed. Hyssop was a very important part of Jewish life. They used this herb on lambs. I used hyssop after Atari taught me about it. I used to make anointing oils out of hyssop. This oil was used for pray-

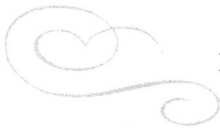

ing and casting out demonic spirits. Also, in the Bible, this oil was used in the synagogue. Hyssop can be mixed with olive oil in the church to anoint people. Some anointing oil consists of frankincense, myrrh, or even hyssop.

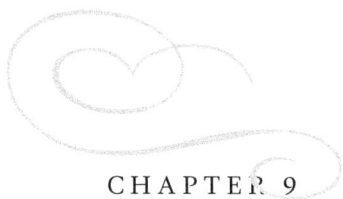

CHAPTER 9

Tsediah
Essential Oil

MAKE TSEDIAH ESSENTIAL OIL
and it is great for skincare. It's good
for someone who suffers from alo-
pecia, eczema, bug bites, snake bites. Lavender
and aloe vera have great skincare properties.
It helps protect and heal the skin. People have
testified that the Tsediah oil left their skin feeling smooth and it keeps it moist. Anyone who
is suffering from bedsores, dry skin, or beginning stages of bedsores. It can help prevent bedsores. I used this oil often and it helps with my
diabetes. Sometimes my skin gets dry and peels.
Especially my feet. I have to moisture my feet
two to three times a day, so my feet won't peel. I

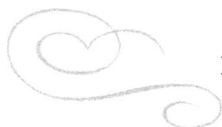

discovered that the sun dries my skin, but the oil helps keep my skin moist.

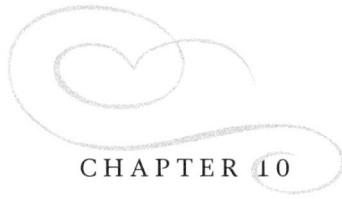

CHAPTER 10

Colunga Oil

COLUNGA OIL IS GOOD for someone who has herpes, chickenpox, muscle spasms, cut, rashes, wounds, burns, skin disease, cold sores. This oil repairs the skin. I also sell salve, which is like a cream so you can rub it into your skin. According to the book, you can drink some calendula oil to help with wounds in the immune systems or hemorrhoids, intestinal diseases, lymphatic system. The calendula stimulates the functioning of the immune system. It helps with swelling. If you drink tea, it can help with menstrual problems and PMS. It helps alleviate the painful side effects of menstruation, such as cramping. It is good for oral health. It has powerful antibacterial properties. It treats gingivitis, plague, oral cavities, or other oral health issues. If you have problems with

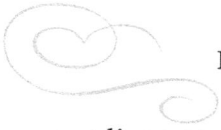

your liver or gall bladder, you can drink it to detox your body. You can use this oil in many ways. It just depends on your symptoms. To drink internally, it has to go through a process and be mixed with glycerin. As a result, a tonic is made, and it must be infused with different oils to digest it. This process involves it sitting for a certain amount of time and being steep and drained. It's not a 1, 2, 3 step. This herb gets rid of stomach issues, especially if you are backed up. If you use the herbs for the outer body compared to the inner body, it has to go through a different process.

CHAPTER 11

Plantain

PLANTAIN HELPS FIGHT AU-TOIMMUNE disorders on the outside of your body. I use plantain for pain, and it's great for chronic pain, especially joint problems such as arthritis. I order my plantain from Star West Botanicals. I used plantain when I made my first herbal salve, and I mixed it with different herbs. Prophetess Yolanda Samuels sent me a testimony about it. Her husband was dealing with pain, and he used it. The herb took away the pain and healed the scab. He used the elderberry blast and the salve of plantain and St. John's. He said the shipping was fast and well secured. They said they highly recommend my products.

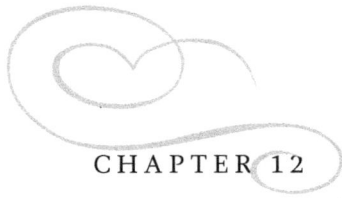

St. John's Wort

S<small>T</small>. J<small>OHN</small>'<small>S</small> <small>WORT</small> <small>HERB</small> can be drunk as tea. It is also known as hypericum perforatum. It is found in North America. The fresh herbs are amazing, and I always order the best quality. It helps with depression and mood disorders such as anxiety and OCD. Plantain can't be drank because it's harmful. However, if someone has bipolar, St. John's may be too potent. St. John's is good for cuts, bruises, sunburns. It contains antibacterial properties. It can be combined with aloe vera and Lavendula. St. John's is fast-acting and can heal the blood and can stop bleeding. It is good for muscle pain, gout, and arthritis. You can also soak your feet in the bath bombs that I make if you are dealing with pain. Next, massage the St. John's salve into your legs. This oil can go in and destroy things that are affecting your body. It helps with hepatitis and shingles. For instance, if they have spots and they get cold, St. John's can help, especially if the tonic is ingested.

Back in the day, they put St. John's in a jar with alcohol and sealed it tight. The alcohol would pull the nutrients out of the herb, and when people would get sick, they would have to drink it. For instance, when bacteria gets on hyssop, it makes penicillin. It goes through a liquefaction process. I used to take penicillin capsules to help with infections. Back in the day, our ancestors didn't go to the doctor, but they went to the garden. The garden brought life and healing because of the plants, herbs, that God created.

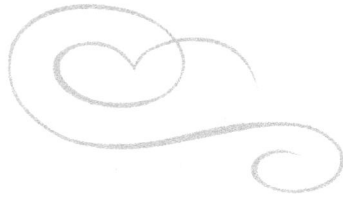

Conclusion

ACCORDING TO WIKIPEDIA, MANDRAKE is an herb from a plant's root found in the Mediterranean and the Himalayas regions. These Mediterranean European mandrakes are perennial herbaceous plants with ovate leaves arranged in a rosette, a thick upright shape, often branched, and bell-shaped flower. The colors are yellow, greenish, and purple berries—the size and shape maximum length is 45 cm (18 in) (Wikipedia.com).

According to Web MD, European Mandrake is an herb subject of many superstitions. Some people believe that it has magical powers. The root and leaves are used to make medicine. The roots are good for treating stomach ulcers, colic, contraception, asthma, hay fever, conversions, arthritis-like pain (rheumatism), and whooping cough. It is also used to reduce certain chemicals that can affect many body systems, such as the eyes, bladder, lungs, bowels, and mouth.

This is what the herbs look like:

It was mind-blowing to learn that the Bible speaks about mandrake. It is written in two places in the Bible: Songs Of Solomon 7:13 and Genesis 30:16. The mandrake gives a smell, and at our gates are all manner of pleasant fruits, new and old which I have laid up for thee, My beloved.

The mandrake was called "Love Flower or Love fruit." Now, as the Shulamite gives a pleasant fruit to my beloved,"' Likewise, Israel will finally give such to Christ Jesus (The Expositor's Study Bible).

Genesis 30:14-17
14 Now Reuben went in the days of wheat harvest and found mandrakes in the field, and brought

them to his mother Leah. Then Rachel said to Leah,
"Please give me some of your son's mandrakes."

¹⁵ But she said to her, "Is it a small matter that
you have taken away my husband? Would you take
away my son's mandrakes also?"

And Rachel said, "Therefore he will lie with you
tonight for your son's mandrakes."

¹⁶ When Jacob came out of the field in the eve-
ning, Leah went out to meet him and said, "You
must come in to me, for I have surely hired you with
my son's mandrakes." And he lay with her that
night.

¹⁷ And God listened to Leah, and she conceived
and bore Jacob a fifth son.

Now, this is one of the herbs that Rachel had
asked her sister Leah to give her so that she may
conceive a man child for Jacob. So this is the
history of increasing sexual healing and fertil-
ization for baby-making. Whatever you need,
God got it. He is the same today, yesterday, and
forevermore.

I will be marketing this product on www.
Misfitforgottens.com and watch God change
and heal many lives as He sees fit. I am not a

doctor, but I know a man with all powers in His hands and His name is JESUS. If it is the Father's will, you will be made whole again. I trust in a God that I knew nothing about because I was not saved, but He Jesus healed my body and made me whole. If He did it for me, He can do it for You.

We must understand that the knowledge and wisdom of the science of herbology have been restricted. Many enemies are out to suppress any legal rights of claiming herbs can be used to be some medicine. In Western culture, herbalists are not to state that these herbs can heal or cure you in any way (Herbs Of Mexico).

The Book of Genesis and many other scriptures talk about the creation of God and how he created every living thing upon this earth. So there's nothing mysterious when it comes down to plants and having the ability to be used for medical use. They've been using it for years and are still using it today. It's just that we may not know exactly what purpose the herbs may be used for. Well, if you're not in the medical field, you may not be able to recognize some of

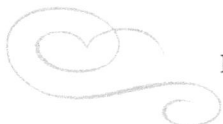

the names of the herbs. The company, Goli, has herbal products such as Ashwagandha, elderberry syrup, Turmeric, etc. and they stated how it is good for the body. Now the world may not realize that these are natural herbs. Knowledge is power and wisdom is the principle of all things; therefore, get and understanding (Proverbs 4:7).

Dr. Edward E. Shook quotes from his book, "I think it is appropriate to explain why herbs are better suited for the treatment of diseases than chemicals and other substances. Herbs are the product of nature and very finely distributed, which are necessary for building up and maintaining the cells of all the organs of the body (Herbs Of Mexico)."

The doctor quotes Ezekiel 47:12, one of my favorite scriptures. *12 And by the river upon the bank thereof, on this side and on that side, shall grow all trees for meat, whose leaf shall not fade, neither shall the fruit thereof be consumed: it shall bring forth new fruit according to his months, because their waters they issued out of the sanctuary: and the fruit thereof shall be for meat, and the leaf thereof for medicine.*

All the laboratories in the world will never be able to imitate the power of God. God's creation aligns with the things we need to support the cells of our bodies and cause the human body to function naturally. Dr. Shooks says, it is true that our bodies contain minerals. They must be obtained from life. Doctor Edward also states plants have the power to take up minerals through their roots from the soil and ASSIMI-LATE and transform them to be utilized as medicine. However, on the other hand, the human body has not the ability to directly assimilate minerals (Herbs Of Mexico).

According to the Journal Of Ethnobiology and Ethnomedicine, all our suggested Biblical Medicinal Plants are known in Ancient Egypt and Mesopotamia. These plants have been in continuous medicinal use in the Middle East down the generations and are being used in the Holy Land today. Precisely in King Solomon's words, *"That which has been is what will be, that which is done is what will be done. And there is nothing new under the sun" (Ecclesiastes 1:9).*

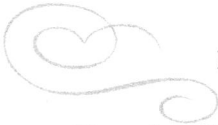

Here is a list of Bible Verses on plants:

Genesis 1:29 (NASB) says, "Then God said behold I have given you every plant yield and see that is on the surface of all the earth, and every tree which has fruits yielding seeds: it shall be full for you."

Genesis 1:11 (NASB) says, "Then said God let the earth sprout vegetation, plants yielding seed, and fruit trees on the earth bearing fruit after their kind with seeds in them, and it was so."

Genesis 9:3 (NASB) says, "Every moving thing that is alive shall be food for you: I have given everything to you, as I gave the green plant."

Psalms 104:14 (NASB) says, "He causes the grass to grow for the cattle and vegetation for the labor of mankind so that they may produce food from the earth."

Genesis 1:12 (NASB) says, "The earth produced vegetation, plants yielding seed according to their kind, and trees bearing fruit with seed in them, according to their kind; and God saw that it was good."

Exodus 12:8 (NASB) says, "They shall eat the flesh that same night, roasted with fire, and they shall eat it with unleavened bread and bitter herbs."

Revelation 22:2 (NASB) says, "in the middle of its street. On either side of the river was the tree of life, bearing twelve kinds of fruit, yielding its fruit every month; and the leaves of the tree were for the healing of the nations."

Hebrews 6:7 (NASB) says, "For ground that drinks the rain which often [a]falls on it and produces vegetation useful to those for whose sake it is also tilled, receives a blessing from God."

Lamentations 3:15 (NASB) says, "He has filled me with bitterness, He has made me drink plenty of wormwood."

Romans 14:2 (NASB) says, "One person has faith that he may eat all things, but the one who is weak eats only vegetables."

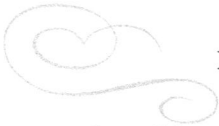

The Bible mentions 128 plants that were part of everyday life in ancient Israel and its Mediterranean neighbors. These plants include almonds, apples, black mustard, cucumber, grapes, mandrake, nettle, poppy, and wormwood.

The migratory patterns of herbs and plants follow those who relied on them. The Levant—which stretches in a crescent around the eastern Mediterranean Sea from Turkey to the Sinai Peninsula and includes modern Syria, Lebanon, Jordan, and Israel—marks the most likely "checkpoint" through which population groups passed as they migrated. As they moved, people carried cuttings, seeds, or saplings of plants and herbs necessary for their well-being or by God's directives.

I pray that God would add a blessing to the reading of this word. May you multiply, replenish, subdue the earth and have dominion. For we are what the word says. We can do what the word says we can do. We have what the word said we can have. We are committed to bring fame to His name and pleasure to His heart. Our Father which art in heaven, hallow be thy name.

Thy Kingdom come; thy will be done on earth as it is in heaven. Give us this day our daily bread and forgive us for our debts as we forgive our debtors. Lead us not into temptation but deliver us all from evil. For thine is the Kingdom, the power, and the glory, forever and ever, Amen.

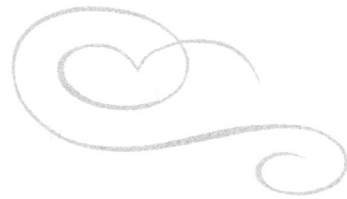

About The Author

STEPHANIE HAM IS THE founder and CEO of Misfits To The Nation, But Chosen By God's Creation. Before marriage, she was known as Stephanie Whack. She is a woman after God's own heart and an intercessor. Stephanie is married to Leo A. Ham. She is a mother of three sons, and four grandchildren: two boys and two girls. She happens to be the #1 Best Seller Book Writing Scribe for The Kingdom. When God called her, He said, "I must work the works of him that sent me, while it is day: the night cometh, when no man can work. As long as I am in the world, I am the light of the world {John 9:4-5}."

Stephanie's favorite Scripture is: "For I know the thoughts that I think toward you, saith the Lord, thoughts of peace, and not of evil, to give you an expected end" (Jeremiah 29:11).

Stephanie's ministry is all about encouraging, uplifting the brokenhearted, hurting, and abused men and women of God. When you're broken from the inside, it's hard to believe in a God who you cannot see. You don't know how He can possibly love someone you... Right? I had to learn that God's Word concerning our lives means so much to Him that He died to save us. Amen. It does not matter to Our Savior if we are a misfit. But what does concerns Him is that we are the core of Jesus's very being. Know that we're Misfits with A Purpose that can change the Nation. God has given Stephanie a keen discernment, intelligence, and a passion for prayer. She loves seeing souls saved. It doesn't matter if you're called an outcast. God loves you. God died for you to live and have life more abundantly.

She has attended the following churches along her Journey:

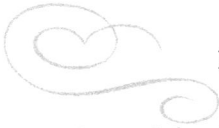

St. Michael's Hope Ministry: Apostle Michael, Prophetess Sharon Woodham CLIO, SC.

Word Of Life Pastor Hodges Bennettsville SC, Solid Rock Holiness: Apostle Ervin Dease and First Lady Mary Dease "aka Spiritual Parents' Bennettsville, SC.

New Creation Christian Church: Bishop Wesley V. Knight & Prophetess Adrian Knight "aka Spiritual Parents" Brooklyn, NY.

The Doors Of Hope: Bishop Michael Blue& First Lady Melinda Blue from Marin SC.

Her educational background consists of the following:

Word Of Life Bible College Studied: The book of Revelation, The Tabernacle, Homiletics. 2002, In Bennettsville SC.

Undergraduate Nyack College study General, Counseling, Abnormal and Child Psychology. Old, New Testament, etc. 2010- 2013

In Manhattan, NY, God started dealing with Stephanie's life and how she felt about herself. She received the vision for her ministry between 2011- 2012 and birthed it out in 2020.

God placed her around people who believed in her and what she couldn't see in herself. God was in the midst the whole time. Nevertheless, everything happens in God's timing

Index

1

1992, 15

A

Abraham, 3
abused, 16, 73
acid reflux, 39
acne, 45
Adam, 2, 3
Aids, 13
alabaster, 22, 25
alcohol, 61
almonds, 10, 70
Aloe Vera, 39
aloes, 23, 26, 40

alopecia, 45, 55

Alzheimer's disease, 32

Amazon, 9, 49

ancestors, 61

animals, 53

Anise, 32, 33, 42, 43, 44

anointing, 24, 53, 54

anthocyanins, 29

antibacterial, 36, 37, 57, 60

anti-inflammatory, 29, 32, 33, 36, 37

anti-microbial, 33, 34

antioxidants, 29

antiseptic, 21, 36

antispasmodic, 21, 36

antiviral, 10, 43, 44

antiviral infections, 10

anxiety, 21, 60

Arabian, 20

aromatherapy, 21

arthritis, 29, 31, 49, 59, 60, 63

Ashwagandha, 66

Asia, 21, 32

Ask A Prepper, 17, 18

asthma, 21, 34, 36, 63

Atara, 9, 10, 11

atherosclerosis, 38

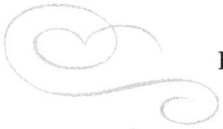

atmosphere, 27

Autoimmune, 32

B

balsam, 23

bath, 43, 44, 60

bathwater, 43

bedsores, 55

beef, 12

Bees, 19

believers, 4, 26

benefits, 1, 4, 19, 32

Bennettsville SC, 74

berries, 29, 62

Bible, 4, 21, 25, 26, 41, 42, 45, 54, 63, 68, 70, 74

big macs, 52

bile-producing, 21

bills, 8

bipolar, 60

birds, 19, 20

Bishop Wesley V. Knight, 74

bitter, 3, 11, 12, 39, 49, 52, 69

Black Jew, 8

bladder, 58, 63

Bladderwrack, 31

blood, 9, 10, 12, 14, 21, 31, 35, 37, 39, 48, 49, 51, 53, 60

blood purifier, 9, 48, 51, 53

blood sugar, 35, 48

blossoms, 48

book, 1, 4, 7, 14, 57, 66, 74

botulism spores, 38

bowel movements, 31

breakfast, 9

breath, 49

broccoli, 10

bronchitis, 21, 34, 36

business, 1, 11, 13, 28

butterfly, 19

C

calcium, 31

cancer, 31, 32, 33, 40, 49

Cannabis, 32

capsules, 9, 50, 61

cassia, 23

cavities, 57

cells, 31, 35, 38, 49, 51, 66, 67

Ceylon, 35, 36

chancre, 12

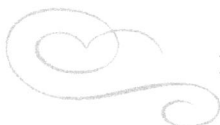

cheesecloth, 43

chemicals, 63, 66

children, 6, 11, 28, 30, 38

Chiropractor, 14

cholesterol, 35, 36, 38, 40

Christians, 1

church, 54

cinnamon, 24, 26, 29, 33, 35, 36, 39, 52

climate, 18, 19, 20

Cloves, 38, 51, 52

coffee, 49

cold, 29, 30, 34, 57, 61

Colunga Oil, 57

congestion, 44

conjunctivitis, 30

copper, 31

cough suppressant, 37

coughs, 29

counterfeit, 4

courtroom, 13

COVID-19, 5

creation, 2, 4, 65, 67

cucumbers, 40

cumin, 33

D

dance, 46

dandelion, 9, 48, 49, 50, 52

Dandelion, 48, 49

Dease, 74

debts, 71

deliverance, 25

demonic, 2, 4, 54

dental, 9

depression, 32, 60

Derek Oldenkamp, 14

detox, 58

devil, 4

devotion, 26

Dewayne Woods, 14

diabetes, 5, 35, 36, 39, 48, 55

diabetic foot ulcers, 37

diarrhea, 35, 43

dictionary, 7

diet, 5, 14

digestion, 32, 43

digestive tract, 31

Dingo, 8

dinner, 9

diseases, 3, 4, 5, 10, 31, 40, 45, 57, 66

disobedience, 3

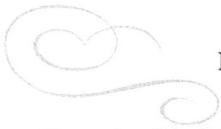

diuretic, 21, 36

doctor, 12, 14, 15, 61, 65, 66

Doctor Josh Axe, 14

Doctor Oz, 14

dominion, 70

douche, 10

Dr. Charles, 14

Dr. Edward E. Shook, 66

Dr. Myles Munroe, 14

Dr. Nicole Aphelian, 20

Dr. Pepe Ramnath, 14

Dr. Pepper, 52

Dr. Rossi Ishmael Khan, 14

Dr. Sebi, 13

drugs, 2

dwarf shrub, 19

E

earth, 2, 6, 65, 68, 70, 71

eat, 2, 5, 9, 10, 12, 26, 49, 52, 69

eczema, 45, 51, 55

Eden, 2, 28

elderberry, 6, 29, 30, 51, 59, 66

Elderberry, 29, 30, 39

Elderberry Blast, 29, 39

emollient, 36

emphysema, 36

enemy, 4

English, 17

Ethnobiology, 67

Ethnomedicine, 67

Europe, 18, 41

Eve, 2, 3

evil, 71, 73

expectorant, 36

eye irritation, 30

Ezekiel, 2, 23, 66

F

Facebook, 14

faucet, 43

fear, 4

feet, 12, 25, 42, 55, 60

fevers, 29

fiber, 31

fire, 47, 69

First Lady Melinda Blue, 74

fish, 10, 40

flower, 18, 30, 37, 42, 49, 62

flowers, 1, 2, 19, 20, 21, 29, 36, 42, 43, 44

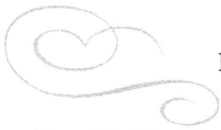

flu, 29, 30, 34, 35, 44

folly, 3

food, 2, 35, 40, 68

fountain, 26

fragrance, 19, 24, 25, 26, 27

France, 17, 18

frankincense, 23, 26, 54

French, 18, 20

fries, 52

fructose, 38

fruit, 2, 26, 32, 63, 66, 68, 69

G

galbanum, 23

gallbladder, 31

garden, 2, 17, 26, 61

Garlic, 40

gastritis, 48

gel, 39

gingivitis, 9, 49, 57

Glory, 13

glucose, 35, 38

glycemic index, 38

glycerin, 58

God, 1, 2, 3, 4, 5, 6, 7, 8, 9, 10, 11, 13, 15, 16, 24, 25, 26, 28, 29, 38, 45, 46, 47, 61, 64, 65, 67, 68, 69, 70, 72, 73, 75
Goli, 6, 66
Gospel singer, 14
grace, 8
Greece, 19
gummies, 6
gums, 39

H

hair, 22, 31
handkerchief, 24
hands, 12, 13, 65
headaches, 21
healthy, 2, 3, 9, 10, 31
heart, 4, 5, 18, 31, 38, 40, 42, 51, 70, 72
heartfelt, 26
heavens, 2
hemorrhoids, 30, 57
hepatitis, 61
herb, 1, 7, 10, 21, 31, 33, 42, 48, 51, 53, 58, 59, 60, 61, 62
herbalist, 1, 9, 15, 50
herbology, 1, 4, 65

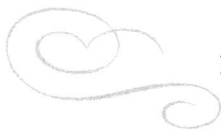

herpes, 37, 57

Herpes, 44

Herpes Simplex I, 44

Himalayas, 21, 62

holistic, 14

Holy Spirit, 8, 13, 26, 27, 46

Honey, 37, 38

Hope, 74

humanity, 5

husband, 1, 59, 64

hypertension, 40, 49

hypocrites, 33

hyssop, 9, 12, 41, 42, 43, 44, 45, 53, 54, 61

Hyssop, 12, 41, 43, 44, 45, 53, 54

I

ice creams, 21

illnesses, 30

immune system, 6, 29, 30, 33, 34, 40, 49, 51, 57

incense, 23, 24

India, 22

infant, 38

infection, 30, 36, 44

infections, 21, 33, 34, 35, 37, 43, 61

inflammation, 31, 33, 34, 45, 49

inflammatory, 31, 33, 34

infusion, 42, 44

insulin, 35, 48

insurance, 14

intercessor, 72

Irish moss, 31

iron, 31

Israel, 28, 41, 63, 70

J

Jacob, 64

jams, 21

Jesus, 4, 16, 26, 27, 40, 47, 53, 63, 65, 73

Jewish, 53

joint pains, 31

Jordan, 70

juice, 36, 39, 48

K

King David, 3, 53

Kingdom, 71, 72

knowledge, 5, 24, 65

L

labor, 68

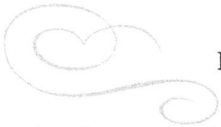

lamb, 3, 10, 12

laryngitis, 36

Lavandula, 17, 18, 19, 20, 21, 24, 25

lavender, 17, 18, 19, 20, 21

Lavender, 18, 21, 45, 55

Leah, 64

leaves, 2, 19, 20, 21, 29, 36, 39, 42, 43, 44, 45, 62, 69

Lebanon, 26, 70

leeks, 40

legacy, 13

leprosy, 42

libido, 11

licorice, 32

lifestyle, 10, 52

lipid, 48

liquefaction, 61

Love, 13, 63

lunch, 9

M

mandrake, 62, 63, 70

Manhattan, NY, 75

Mary, 11, 25, 26, 74

meal, 9, 35, 38, 39

meat, 3, 12, 66

medicine, 1, 2, 12, 24, 40, 62, 65, 66, 67

Mediterranean, 17, 18, 20, 62, 70

melons, 40

memory, 26

menopause, 51

mercy, 8, 33

Mesopotamia, 67

metabolism, 31, 35

Michael, 74

minerals, 31, 67

mint, 17, 33, 42

miscarriages, 11

Misfits Forgotten, 1

mold, 12

molested, 16

mollusks, 24

money, 2, 6

monitor, 38

mood disorders, 60

mouthwash, 39

movie, 13

mucus, 44

Mullein, 36

muscle spasms, 37, 57

muscle sprains, 30

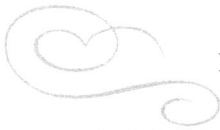

myrrh, 23, 26, 36, 40, 54

N

nails, 31
Nard, 21
national board, 15
nations, 5, 69
nerve damage, 14
Nerve Neuropathy, 14
New Testament, 74
Nicodemus, 40
North America, 9, 48, 60
nursing field, 12
nutrients, 61

O

oatmeal, 10
Obadiah, 11
obesity, 10
OCD, 60
oils, 1, 36, 45, 53, 58
ointment, 22
Old Testament, 53
olive oil, 54

onions, 40

onycha, 24

outcast, 73

P

Pacific Botanicals, 50

pain, 4, 21, 29, 31, 32, 33, 36, 39, 42, 45, 59, 60, 63

pain relief, 21

palmar lesion, 12

pancreas, 48

pandemic, 5

passion, 28, 73

Passover, 3, 12

Paul, 24, 25

paycheck, 8

payment plan, 14

penicillin, 12, 61

perfume, 21, 22, 25

perseverance, 46

petals, 19

Pharisees, 33

pharmaceutical industry, 5, 6, 15

phytochemicals, 32, 33

plague, 57

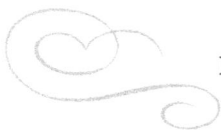

Plantain, 59, 60

plants, 1, 2, 5, 6, 25, 26, 48, 61, 62, 65, 67, 68, 70

poem, 25

poison ivy, 44

pollen, 37

pomegranates, 26

pores, 51

pork, 12

powder, 9, 50

Power, 13, 30

praise, 47

prayer, 25, 73

pregnant, 11, 29

Prophetess Adrian Knight, 74

Prophetess Yolanda Samuels, 59

prosper, 5

psoriasis, 37

purify, 3, 10

R

raisins, 10

raped, 16

rashes, 57

red clover, 9, 51, 52

red meats, 10

Red Sea, 24

refrigerator, 29

regimen, 1, 9, 10, 11, 15

remission, 15

research, 12, 21, 30

respiratory, 21, 32, 34

revelation, 4, 47

ringworms, 45

river, 2, 66, 69

rolled oats, 10

rose hip, 29

S

salads, 10, 52

salvation, 7

Sarah, 3

Sarsaparilla, 31

Satan, 4

Savior, 73

scabs, 4

scars, 4, 45

scribes, 33

Sea moss, 31

season, 29, 46

sex drive, 11

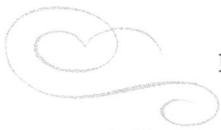

sexual disease, 16

Sharon, 74

shingles, 61

Shulamite, 63

sick, 1, 3, 15, 34, 61

sickness, 9

skin, 31, 37, 39, 43, 44, 45, 51, 55, 56, 57

smoothies, 1

snow, 53

Solomon, 23, 25, 26, 27, 63, 67

sores, 12, 57

Soursop, 31

soymilk, 10

Spain, 17, 18, 19

spices, 23, 24, 26, 36

Spikenard, 21, 24, 26

spirit, 43

sponge, 53

Sprite, 52

St. John's Wort, 60

St. Mary's hospital, 11

stacte, 24

Star West Botanicals, 50, 59

STD, 3, 12, 53

Stephanie, 72, 73, 75

steward, 5

stomach, 58, 62

stress, 21

stripper, 8

strokes, 5

sugar, 8, 35, 37, 38, 39, 48, 49

sugar daddy, 8

summer, 18, 20

sunburn, 39

supernatural, 2

superstitions, 62

surgery, 6

sweet potatoes, 10

sweetener, 42

symptoms, 4, 13, 15, 16, 29, 51, 58

Syphilis, 8, 10

Syria, 70

T

Tabitha Brown, 6

tea, 9, 21, 29, 30, 34, 35, 42, 43, 44, 49, 50, 52, 57, 60

teeth, 9, 18, 49, 50

temple, 8, 27

temptation, 71

The Lost Book Of Herbals Remedy, 35, 38

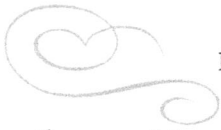

therapy, 30

tincture, 21, 29, 33

tongue, 12

tonic, 10, 42, 58, 61

tracheitis, 36

treatments, 15

trees, 2, 5, 26, 66, 68

trials, 46

tribulations, 46

triglycerides, 35, 38

Tsediah, 45, 55

tub, 43

tuberculosis, 36

turkey, 10

Turmeric, 31, 66

turnips, 49

U

unleavened bread, 69

urinary tract, 21, 34, 35

V

vaginal opening, 12

vinegar, 21, 53

virus, 14, 30, 36, 44

vision, 75

vitamins, 31

voice, 15

W

walnuts, 10

wart, 36

whooping cough, 63

wind, 26

womb, 15

women, 10, 29, 73

world, 13, 26, 66, 67, 72

wormwood, 69, 70

worship, 24

wounds, 3, 37, 39, 43, 57

Y

Yellow dock, 31

Z

zinc, 31

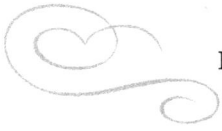

www.ingramcontent.com/pod-product-compliance
Lightning Source LLC
Chambersburg PA
CBHW060248030426
42335CB00014B/1625